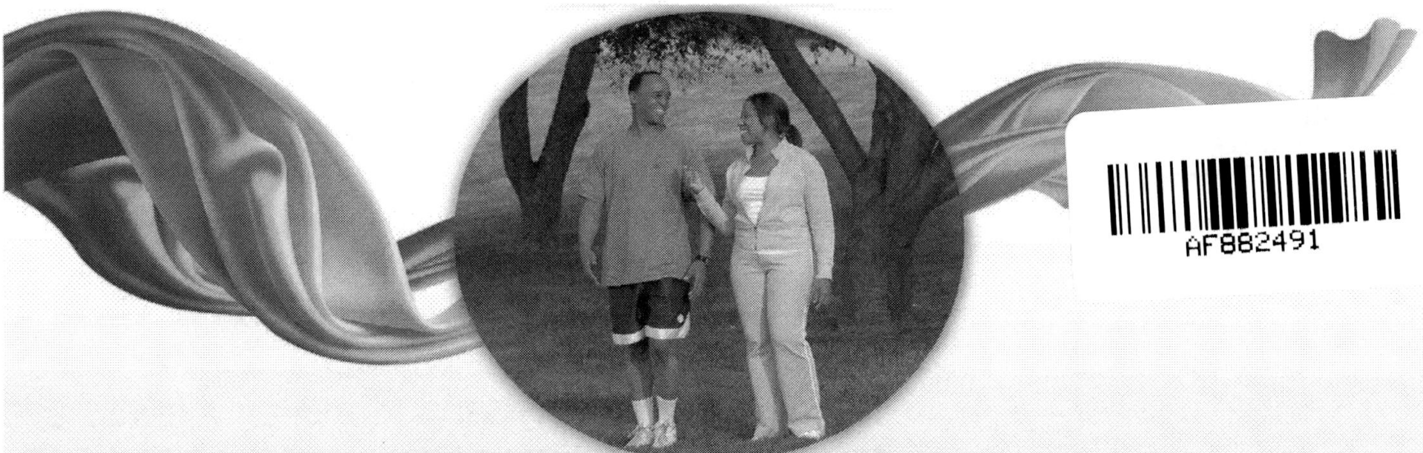

Keys To Virility & Vitality

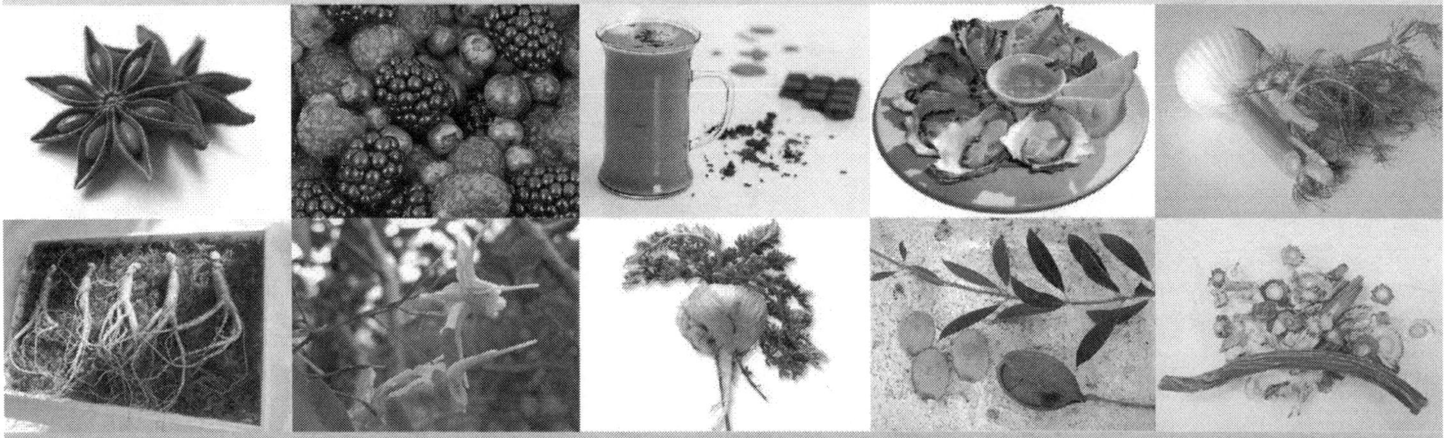

ELLEN KAMHI, Ph.D, R.N., AHG, AHN-BC
The Natural Nurse®
naturalnurse.com

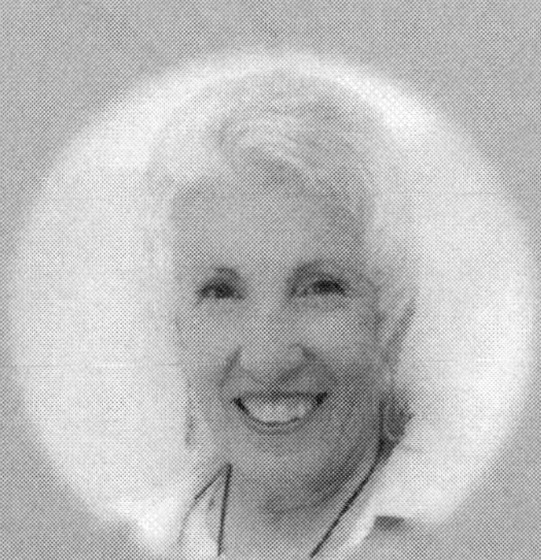

$9.95
ISBN 978-0-9723204-3-6
50995>
9 780972 320436

ISBN: Ebook 978-0-9723204-3-6

Rev. Date: 1/1/2016

Author Contact:
Ellen Kamhi PhD, RN, AHG, AHN-BC
www.naturalnurse.com
www.facebook.com/NaturalNurse
✆: 800-829-0918

Natural "Aphrodisiacs" for Men and Women

Foods and herbs can be very safely and effectively used to boost virility and vitality! Some of these substances have undergone scientific scrutiny, and the 'hows' and 'whys' of their enhancing nature are now understood. Others have stood the test of time afforded by long time traditional use.

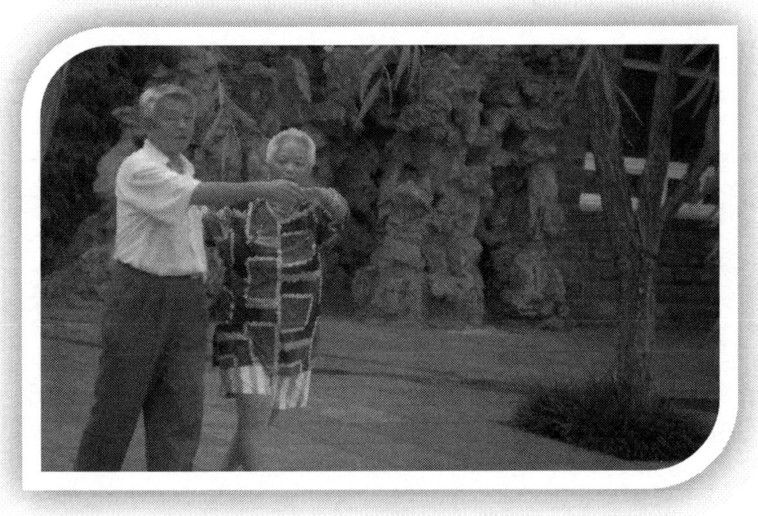

Aging Gracefully, or Healthy Aging, includes slowing down the signs and symptoms that occur as people get older. Healthy Aging focuses on increasing overall feelings of health and wellness, into the golden years. The best way to do this (beyond being blessed with longevity genes) is to eat small meals of mostly organic vegetables and small amounts of high quality protein, drink clean water, and include moderate exercise and stress reduction techniques in your daily routine. Particular foods and herbs can also be useful. These natural substances have a long history of use as Aphrodisiacs, but along with their ability to boost libido, they also support overall virility and vitality!

The dictionary definition of Aphrodisiac is: something that arouses or intensifies sexual desire. The word probably originated in the early 18th century, gleaned from the Greek, *Aphrodisiakos*- arousing sexual desire, and *Aphrodite*-the goddess of love.

Humankind's quest for substances that increase both the pleasure and potency of sexual encounters spans the ages. In civilizations past and present high honors and awards have been given to 'healers' (or drug companies) who have been able to produce effective sexual stimulants. Tribal medicine men and women would constantly experiment with plants, gemstones and animal parts in search of potency elixirs. Cave drawings, and ancient manuscripts describe all manner of herbs, teas and potions that have been used for their true or imagined erotic enhancement potential.

A few natural substances have been scientifically proven to do this on a consistent basis. Most supposed aphrodisiacs actually act as tonics, increasing virility over time, usually by supplying nutrients which feed the glands and organs. Others may relate to psychological and mind/body interactions.

FOOD

The Encyclopedia Britannica says the following in reference to the stimulating nature of food:

> *... The combination of various sensuous reactions - the visual satisfaction of the sight of appetizing food, the olfactory stimulation of their pleasing smells and the tactile gratification afforded the oral mechanism by rich, savory dishes - tend to bring on a state of general euphoria conducive to sexual expression.*

A wide variety of foods have been used for their virility properties. People often viewed the 'seed quality' of a food, such as eggs or bulbs to be indicative of their highly energetic nature, since they contain the 'seed of life'. Food with a natural phallic shape, such as carrots or asparagus, were also thought to have enhancement value. It is interesting to note that many foods thought to be aphrodisiacs by the ancients, are actually high in nutrients that are needed for the effective function of organs and glands, and they prove to be especially effective if a person is low in those nutrients.

Unfortunately, the standard western diet of highly processed 'junk food' is linked to obesity and almost every degenerative illness known. The same nutrient rich, naturally based diet that protects the body from the ravages of disease, will also enhance the function of all the glands and ensure the production of adequate hormone levels to maintain vitality and virility into advanced age. The fact is, people who eat a diet high in organic vegetables, and foods rich in Omega 3 oils and other essential fatty acids, such as nuts and seeds, along with maintaining a daily exercise regimen, and having a strong association of social interactions, are the most likely candidates to experience a longer healthier life.

Here is a listing of several foods that have gained a reputation as virility and vitality enhancers:

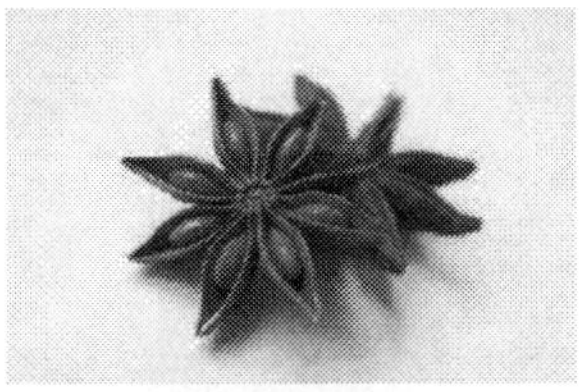

Anise: Anise is a licorice scented spice with a seed pod that is in the perfect shape of a star. The Greeks and Romans used is an aphrodisiac by sucking on the seeds directly, or brewing them as a tea.

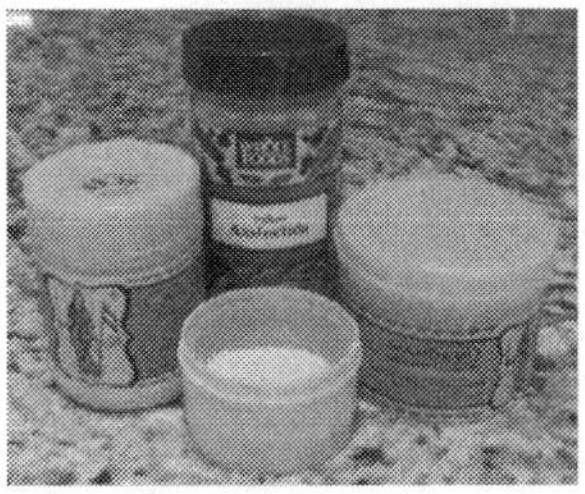

Asafoetida: is prepared from a plant with exotic names, such as 'devil's dung', which probably refers to the strange odor (from the latin '*foetidus*' for stinking), and strong, garlic-like, taste of this Indian herb. It has been used to relieve digestive disorders, as well as a mild laxative and sexual stimulant in Ayurvedic medicine from India for centuries.

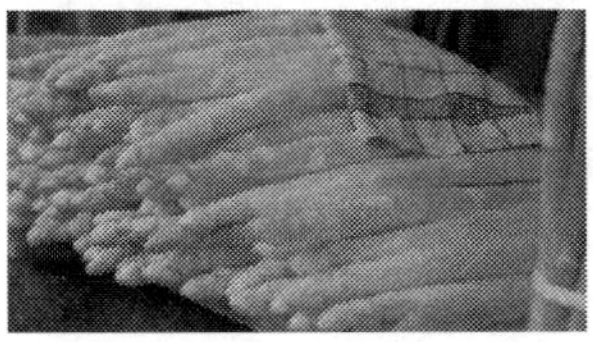

Asparagus: Asparagus is obviously a 'phallic food'. Asparagus is considered a food that dispels anger, in Traditional Chinese Medicine. Steam asparagus, and share a shaft with your lover. Its rich Vitamin E content is also sex healthy and supports vitality and virility!

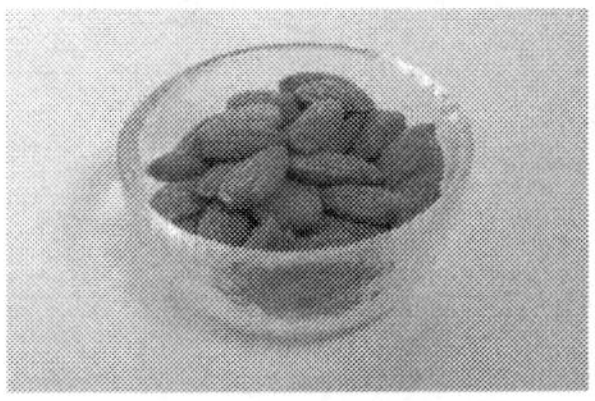

Almond: The aroma of almond has been used to heat up a bed chamber in many societies. Almond paste (marzipan), can be used as an edible love potion, and enhances the level of healthy nutrients such as magnesium and Omega 3 fatty acids.

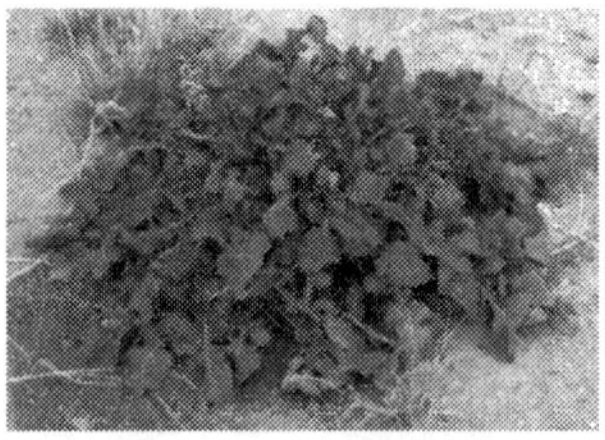

Arugula: The bitter taste of arugula releases digestive enzymes that allow the body to absorb the micronutrients the body needs for high level health. This vegetable has been touted for its aphrodisiac properties since the first century AD. Combine arugula into a paste with pine nuts, pistachios and basil for a vitality enhancing pesto sauce.

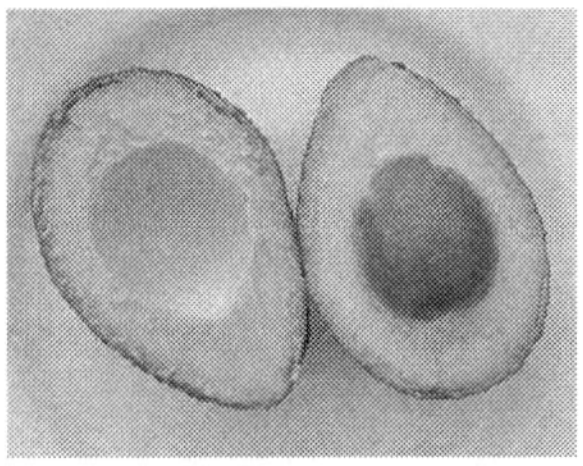

Avocado: Just picture a large ripe green avocado, and you can imagine why the Aztecs called the avocado tree *Ahuacuati,* which means testicle tree. Avocados are a great source of the 'good oils' needed for the production of sex hormones in both men and women.

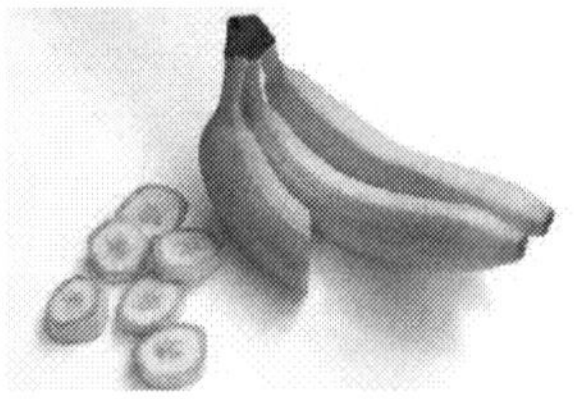

Banana: Bananas are one of the most outwardly phallic fruits. In addition to the common yellow banana, those who have visited the Caribbean may have seen the flower on a banana tree- it also has a very strong vitality overtone. Bananas are high in potassium and other vitamins and minerals used by the body to build sex hormones.

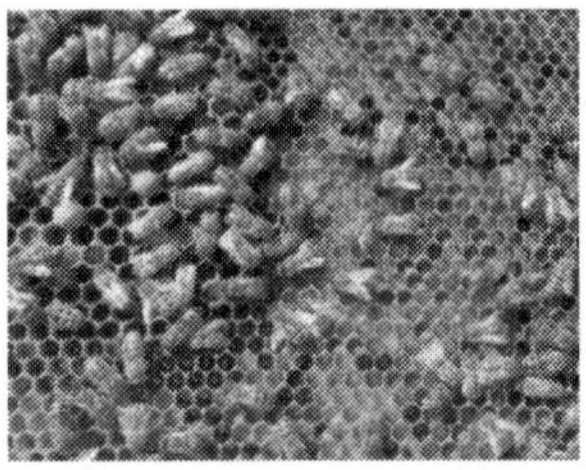

Bee Pollen: This bee product is actually the male sex cell of flowers collected by bees, which pollinates the female flower parts. Bee pollen is extremely high in nutrition, and is truly an anti-aging super-food with over 185 nutrients. It increases overall vitality, virility and energy. Try a small amount at first. People with pollen allergies may be sensitive to bee pollen.

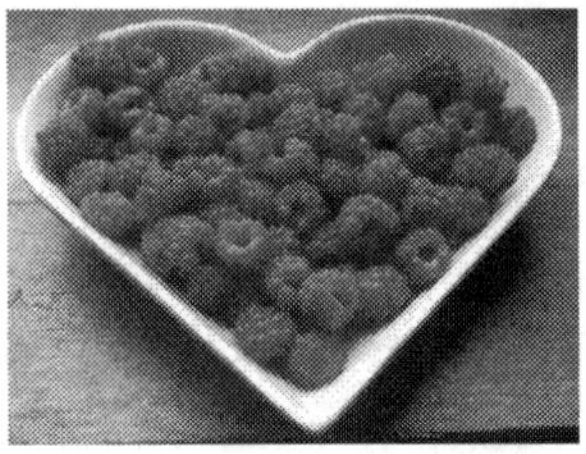

Berries: Sweet juicy strawberries and raspberries are often associated with ripe youthful energy. Berries are actually the seed containing fruits that contain the plants life force energy. Berries are high in bioflavonoids and vitamin C, which heighten health, energy and vitality.

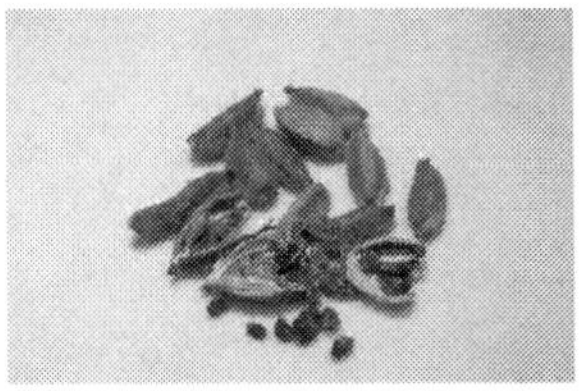

Cardamom: Cardamom is an Indian spice, used to help circulation and blood flow to all areas of the body. One ancient remedy suggests a 'cure' for impotence by gently boiling 3 cardamom pods in one cup of milk for five minutes. Then add one teaspoon of honey. This will spice up your love life!

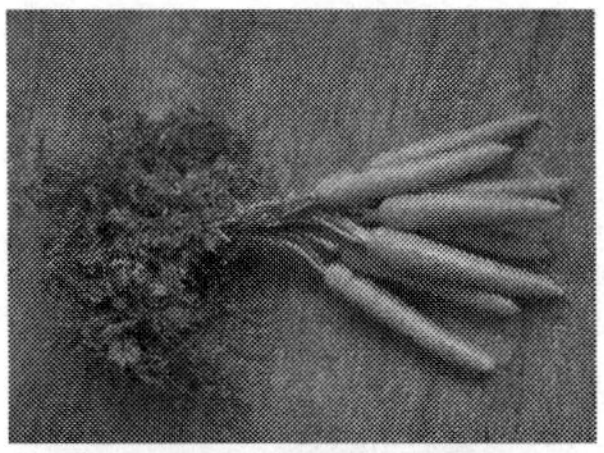

Carrot: Carrots are highly nutritious, and are full of mixed carotenoids, needed by the body for gland health, as well as the well known healthy effects for the eyes and circulatory support. Excellent to include in your vitality and virility program.

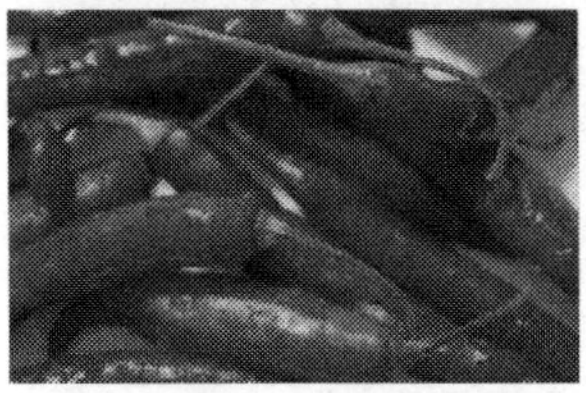

Cayenne: A constituent known as capsaicin, stimulates nerve endings and adds to the 'heat' that cayenne is well known for. It raises the pulse and increases circulation to all areas of the body.

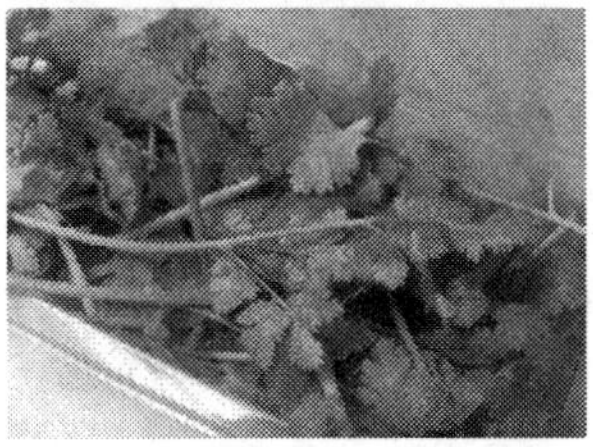

Celantro: This dark green vegetable produces the seed, Coriander that is used as a spice. Both Coriander and Celantro have been used for their aphrodisiac qualities for at least 1000 years before it was mentioned in "The Arabian Nights". Celantro is high in vitamins and minerals, and there is some evidence that it can 'chelate' negative heavy metals from the body.

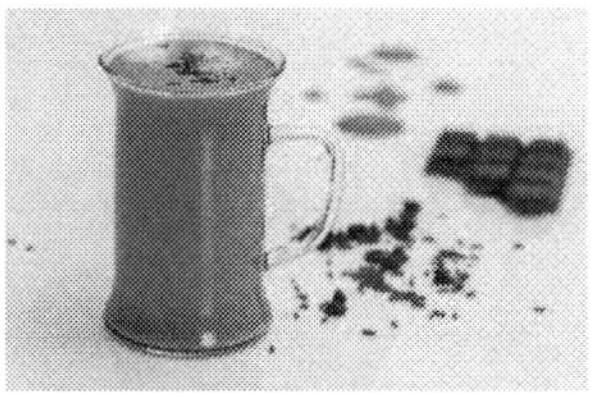

Chocolate: Chocolate is the treat most often associated with love and romance. Its rich sensuous nature, and 'melt in your mouth' texture is one of life's hedonistic pleasures. It has been used by ancient civilizations such as the Aztecs who called it 'food of the Gods'. Chocolate is high in magnesium and other minerals, and contains a compound called phenylethylamine, the feel good 'love chemical'. It is found in high levels in people who are 'in love'.

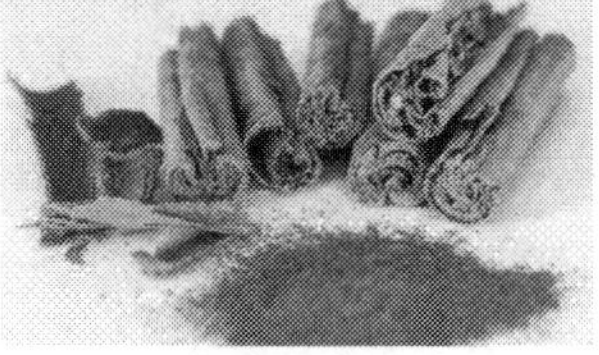

Cinnamon: The distinctive aroma of cinnamon evokes a strong romantic response in both men and women. Cinnamon helps to balance blood sugar and aids in the maintenance of high level of energy, vitality and virility! Both its scent and flavor helps to set a romantic mood.

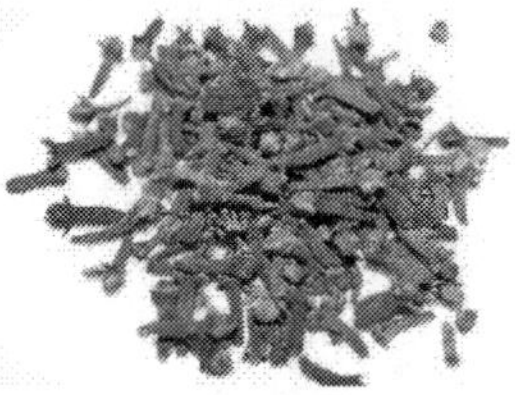

Cloves: have a long history of medicinal use, and remain an herbal analgesic treatment for toothaches to this day. Cloves contain chemical constituents that cause a pleasant numbing of nerve endings, and have been used as an aphrodisiac spice since the third century BC in China. In the Netherlands, several medieval herbalists touted the sexual powers of cloves, indicating that drinking clove tea along with milk will support a healthy virility response.

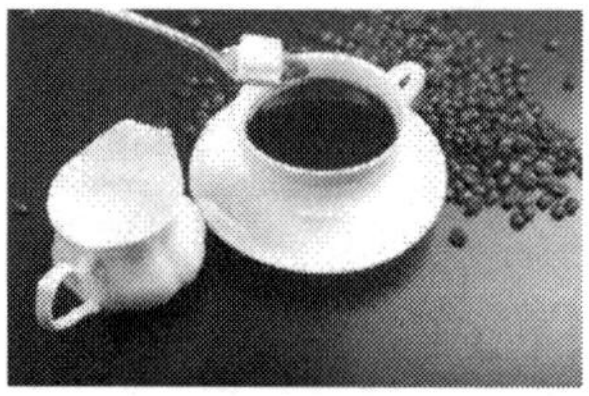

Coffee: The rich warm flavor of coffee is a hedonistic delight, especially when it is enhanced with exotic additives like hazelnut and vanilla. Coffee contains caffeine, a stimulant well known to make you want to 'get and and go'. (Too much, though, can ware out the adrenal glands and interfere with sustained energy)

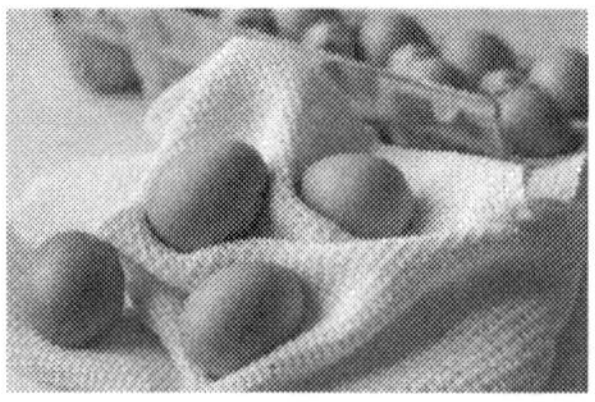

Eggs: Eggs were believed to help alleviate many low energy ailments in countries as diverse as Egypt, China and Europe. The egg is a natural sex aid on many levels. Obviously it is, in itself a sex cell, that harbors the beginning of life. Egg shaped stones are used in 'tantra' to exercise the sexual organs. Eggs are high in complete protein, Vitamins A and B-12, and most of the minerals required by the body, such as iodine, phosphorus, zinc and selenium.

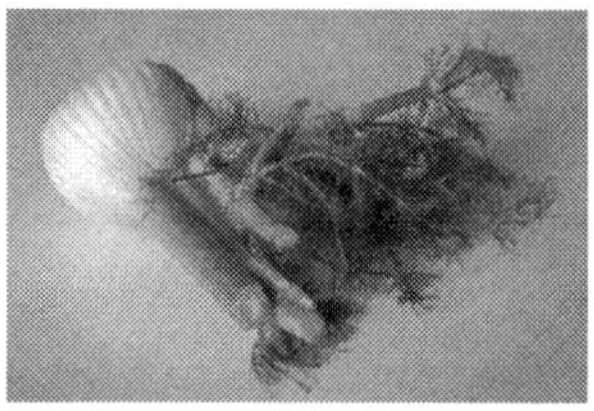

Fennel: The licorice flavor and bulbous nature of fennel, along with the elongated stalk, have sustained its use as an erotic vegetable since ancient Egypt. In the 1930's scientists considered using fennel as a source of estrogen since it contains estragole, an estrogen like substance. Research has proven a libido enhancing effect in rats. It's a delicious vegetable to add to your vitality and virility program.

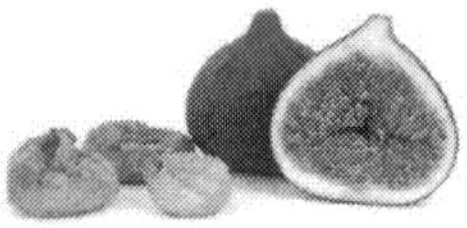

Figs: Figs are high in vitamin A, potassium and calcium, and boast the highest mineral content of all common fruits. Research performed by Rutgers University in New Jersey has determined that dried figs contain Omega-3 and Omega-6 essential fatty acids, as well as a number of phytosterols, needed by the body for sex hormone production and healthy glandular activities.

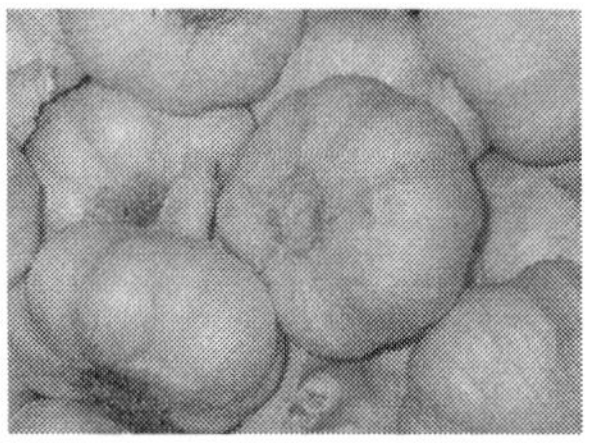

Garlic: Garlic has traditionally been used in civilizations worldwide for its health enhancing properties. Modern science collaborates its benefits for cardiovascular wellness. Indian spiritual traditions insist that yogis, who wish to be celibate, refrain from consuming garlic, which increases 'heat' to the genital areas.

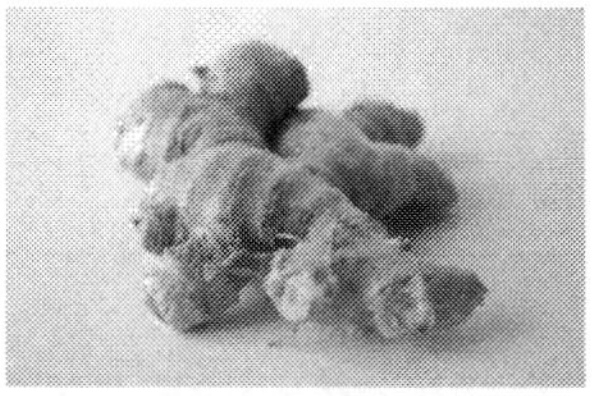

Ginger: The hot spicy taste of ginger is a stimulant for circulation to all the organs, and has anti-inflammatory qualities that can soothe aches and pains, when used both internally and as a topical agent. Ginger can be made into a tea for drinking, and used as a hot compress on achy areas of the body. It can really 'spice up' your love life.

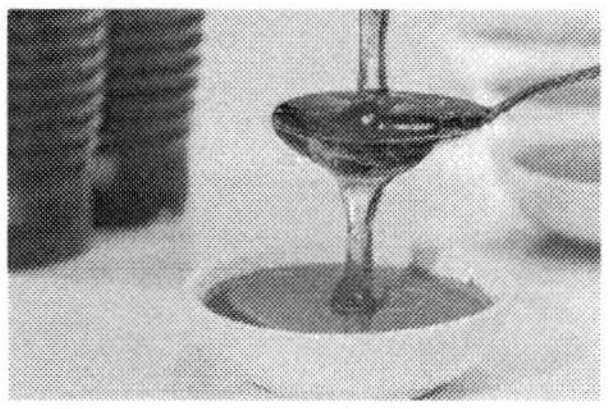

Honey: Honey has been used since ancient Egyptian times to correct impotence. The tradition of the "Honeymoon" refers to the use of Mead, a fermented drink made from honey, by both partners on the first night of their marriage to relieve first time anxiety, and begin nuptial bliss on a sweet note. No reason why seniors can't take advantage of this mixture for vitality and virility!

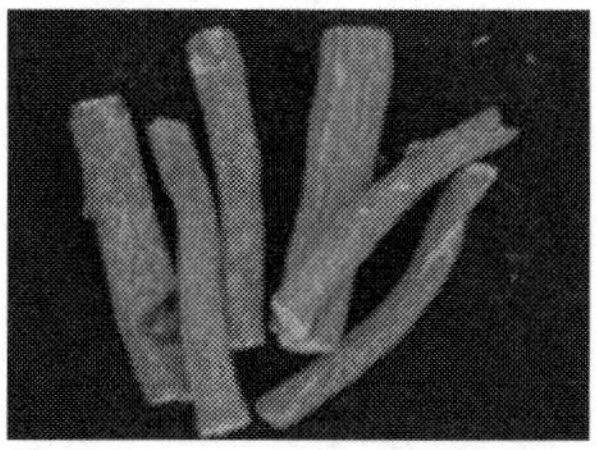

Licorice: Licorice root provides a unique sweet, sensuous flavor. It has long been favored for its love and lust enhancing properties in traditional folklore. Licorice root contains compounds needed for the formation of female sex hormones, and supports the adrenal glands in men and women, important for strength, energy, virility and vitality. The Smell and Taste Foundation in Chicago has discovered that woman find the smell of licorice an erotic stimulant.

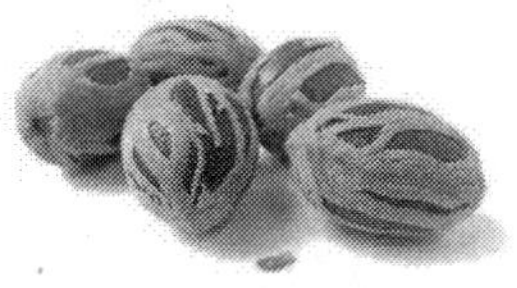

Nutmeg: Nutmeg can be a dangerous hallucinogen if used in high quantities, but is a stimulating spice when sprinkled with a light touch. It was used by Arabs, Greeks, Romans and Hindus for its virility effects, and was prized by Oriental woman for this purpose. Nutmeg contains myristicin, a chemical similar to the hallucinogen mescalin. One recipe calls for crushing a boiled egg along with honey and nutmeg, and eating it ½ hour before romantic activities.

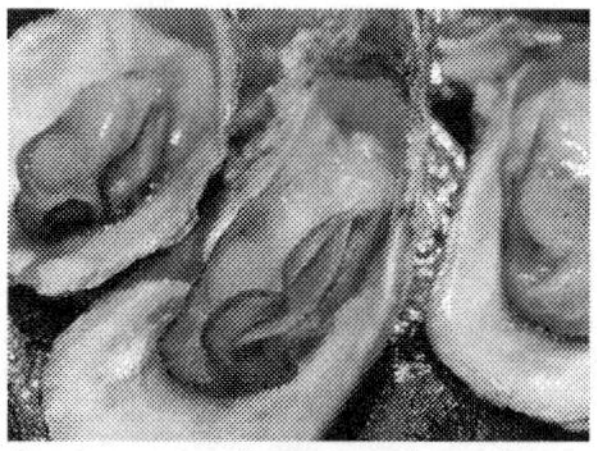

Oyster: Oysters enjoy a long history as an aphrodisiac. Aphrodite, the Greek Goddess of Love, is often pictured springing out of the sea on an oyster shell. Romans documented the oyster as an aphrodisiac, especially because it was considered to look like female genitalia. Oysters are high in protein and minerals such as iodine, phosphorus and zinc. Zinc is particularly important because it is linked to hormone production and utilization.

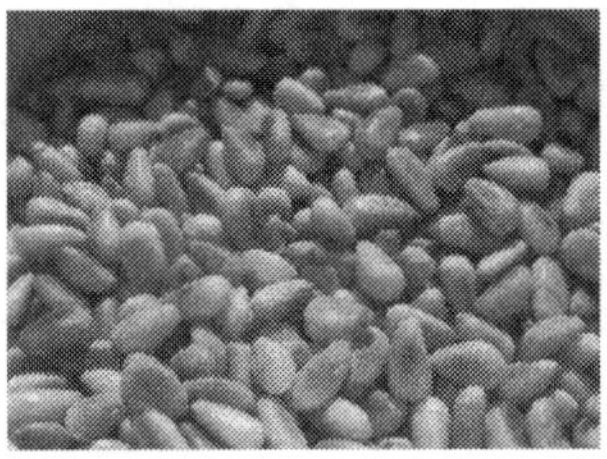

Pine Nuts: Pine nuts have been employed since medieval times as a libido stimulant, as described in the medieval medical manuscript, "*Tacuinum Sanitatis in Medicina*". The Greek physician, Galen, wrote in the 2nd Century A.D., that a mixture of honey, almonds and pine nuts eaten before bed for three nights, will increase a man's virility. The roman poet Ovid, includes pine nuts in his poem "*Ars Amatoria*", "The Art of Love". Pine nuts are also called "pignoli" nuts and are often used in Pesto recipes. They are very high in zinc, the 'love' mineral.

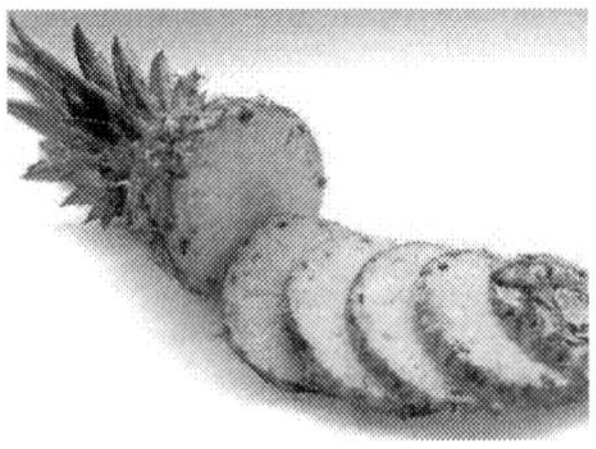

Pineapple: The flamboyant pineapple has been used as a symbol for opulence and glamour for centuries. It often graced bedposts as a decorative addition to 'juice up' the marriage bed. Pineapple juice is believed to sweeten seminal fluids, and is included as a treatment for impotence in homeopathic medicine.

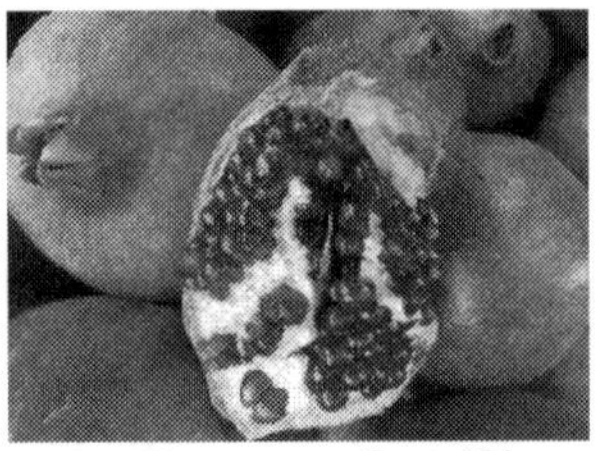

Pomegranate: The pomegranate has been called the "Love Apple" and has a long history as a sexual symbol. The goddess of Love, Aphrodite, supposedly planted it on Cyprus as a gift to lovers. When a pomegranate is cut open, it resembles an ovary full of seeds, and was eaten by both sexes to enhance fertility and virility. In addition to high levels of Vitamin C and potassium, pomegranates contain a form of estrogen called estrone.

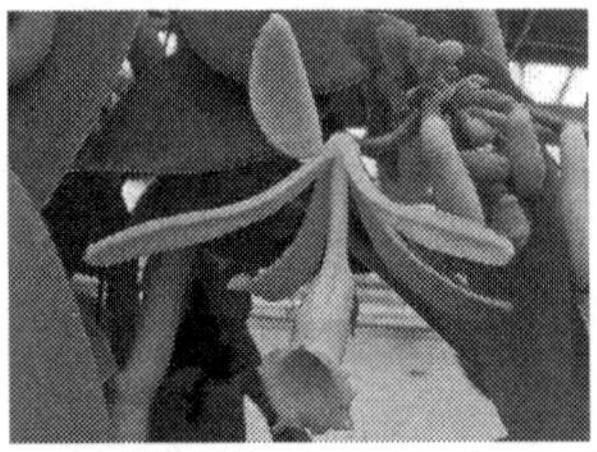

Vanilla: The long vanilla bean is suggestive of a phallic shape, while the name of this lush flavoring spice is derived from the same root word as 'vagina'. The bean is the dried fruit of the orchid, *Vanilla planifolia*, which also visually mirrors female genitalia. The warm, rich scent and taste of vanilla is associated with love and lust. The medical book, *Swedish pharmacopoedia* (1849) recommended vanilla as an aphrodisiac acting through its aroma as much as through its taste.

Recipes For Virility and Vitality

Here are a few recipes that have had tried and true success. Remember that the mood and mode are just as important as the ingredients. As you prepare the meal, visualize the intended outcome. Infuse the ingredients with the intention of your desire. You will not be disappointed!

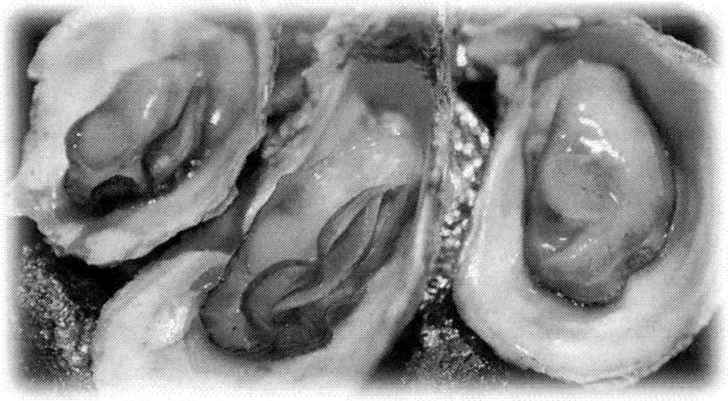

Oysters on the ½ shell

Split Raw Oysters on a decorative plate

Have sliced lemons, limes and cayenne hot sauce available

Feed each other the 'slippery' oysters

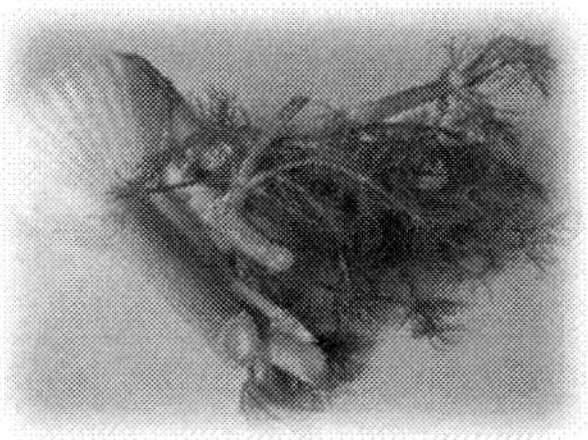
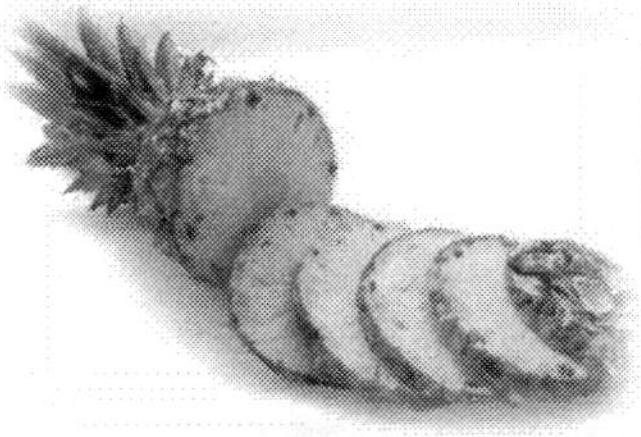
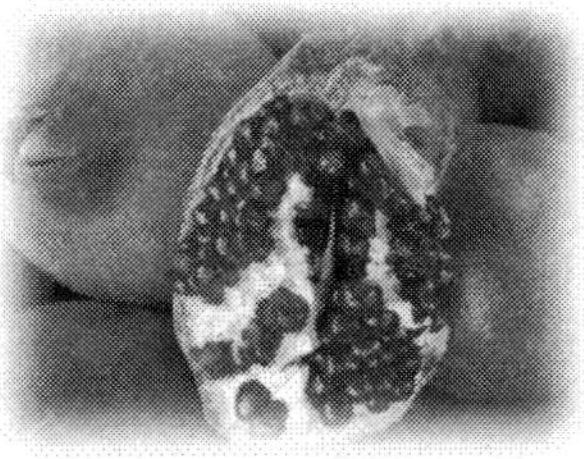
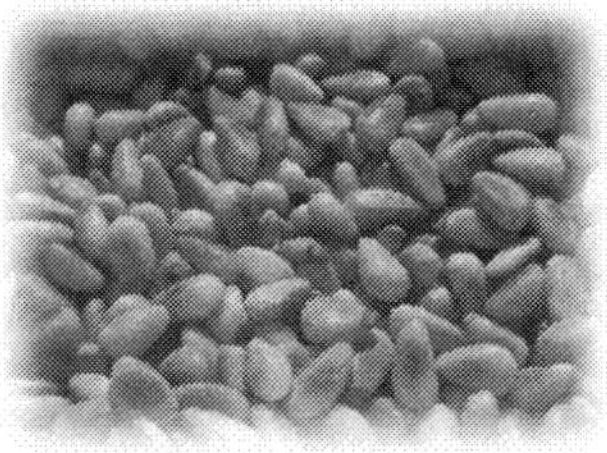

Fennel, Pineapple, Pomegranate and Pine Nut Salad

1 fennel bunch, thinly sliced stalks and bulb

1 pineapple, sliced into bite size pieces-skin removed

20 pine nuts

15 mint leaves

1 whole pomegranate

In a medium size salad bowl, combine cut up fennel and pineapple slices. Scoop all the red seed pods out of the pomegranate and mix them into the bowl. Sprinkle the pine nuts and mint leaves on top of the mixture. Serve within one hour of preparation.

(You will need an extra bowl to 'spit out' the pomegranate seeds, after sucking off the red juice.)

Aphrodisiac Smoothie

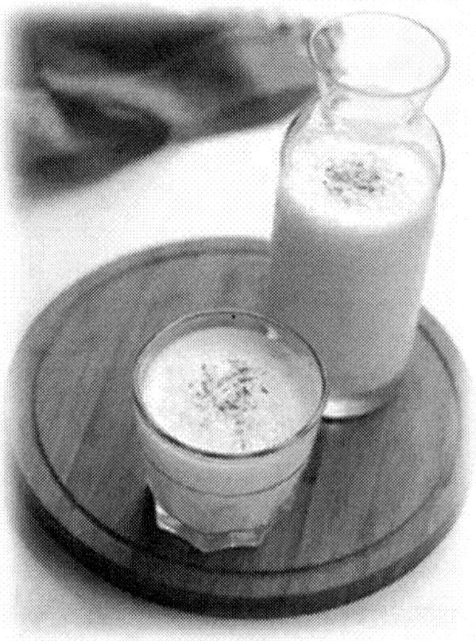

1 cup Organic Vanilla Soy Milk or Rice Milk

2 Cloves

1 Cardamom Pod

1 Cinnamon Stick

1 banana

2 ice cubes

½ cup Organic Vanilla Yogurt

Blend all ingredients in a blender; share with a lover!

HERBS

Woman and men throughout the ages have experimented with various plant substances in an endless search for useful aphrodisiacs that support virility and vitality. Many folkloric tales are linked to elixirs derived from plants. Although some of these stories are simply 'old wives tales', those old wives may well have held the knowledge that kept them happy and healthy into advanced years. There are many herbs that have stood the test of time in recognition of their ability to stimulate and sustain vibrancy over a lifespan into advanced age.

Here are some of the herbs that both ancient shamans and modern scientists credit with healthy aging. Some of these herbs have been studied scientifically. Many others have a long history of traditional use, although they have not as yet been put to the test by the 'gold standard of science'. Dosage recommendations are for a normal 150 pound person, and may vary greatly. Cautions reflect specific known health problems that have been associated with a particular herb. If we write ' no known adverse effects', it means none are known at the time this book was written, but does not guarantee safety for a given individual. As with all nutritional therapies, do not use any of these while pregnant, nursing or taking prescription medications without the advice of your health care practitioner.

Damiana (*Turnera aphrodisiaca, diffusa)*

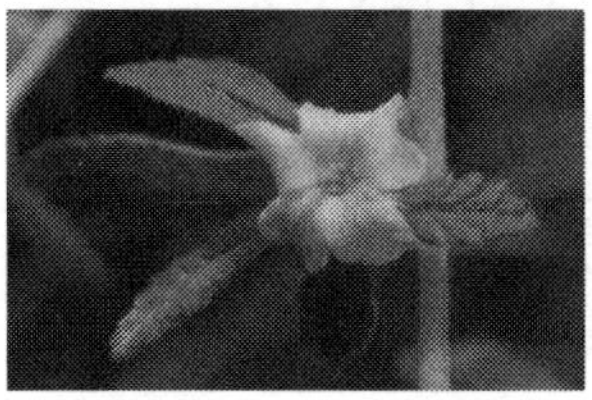

The leaves of the shrub of the Damiana plant has a long history of use as an herbal medicine in Mexico, dating back to the ancient Aztec and Mayan civilizations. Along with other chemical constituents, Damiana contains beta-sitosterol, a phytosterol that may be involved with its effects on the virility. Damiana is a helpful tonic for the nervous system, the genitourinary tract, and the kidneys, and is used for its abilities to tone the mucous membranes of the reproductive organs. The species name of Damiana- "aphrodisiaca", refers to the most renowned use of this herb, as an aphrodisiac and sexual stimulant for both sexes. Damiana was listed in the National Formulary from 1888-1947, and was recommended by physicians for menstrual difficulties including headache, acne, insufficient flow, delayed menstruation in adolescent girls, irritability and lack of sexual desire. In Jamaican folk medicine, it is called *Ram Goat Dash Along*, because when male goats eat it, their libido increases dramatically! Shamans have used damiana during rituals because it helped to break inhibitions and promote the feeling of 'astral travel' to explore spiritual dimensions.

Dosage: Tea- add 1 tsp crushed or powdered leaf to 1 cup hot water-steep for 10 - 15 min., Drink 2-3 cups/day
Tincture/Extract- 10- 20 drops 3 times/day
Capsules- 300-500 mg 3 times/day

Cautions: No cautions have been noted for the use of this herb, except a slight laxative effect

Deer Antler

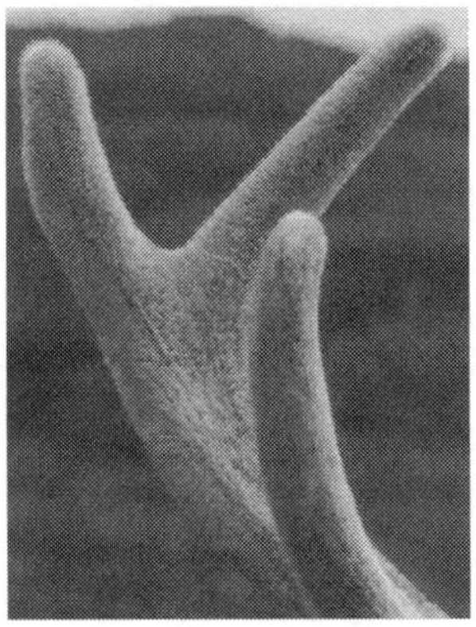

Deer Antler is not an herb, but an animal part, that has been prized in Chinese medicine as a vitality stimulant for centuries. A silk scroll was discovered in a Chinese tomb which describes the use of deer antler as a remedy for over 50 illnesses. It is considered one of the strongest 'yang' tonics. The antlers are harvested without harm to the animals, since they shed their antlers naturally. Scientific studies show that deer antler is useful for anemia, by increasing hemoglobin, as well as the number of red blood cells. In women deer antler increases the strength of contraction and tone of the uterus, which can lead to increased orgasmic intensity. It has an adaptogenic effect, which enhances overall strength and endurance, and decreases fatigue. Current research is linking the use of the velvet scraped off deer antler to beneficial effects such as increased testosterone level, cartilage growth and repair, blood pressure and cholesterol balancing, enhanced immune function, and a decrease in stress related illness.

Dosage: 500mg-1000 mg/ day

Cautions: There are no known adverse effects related to the use of this supplement

Fenugreek (*Trigonella Foenum-Graceum)*

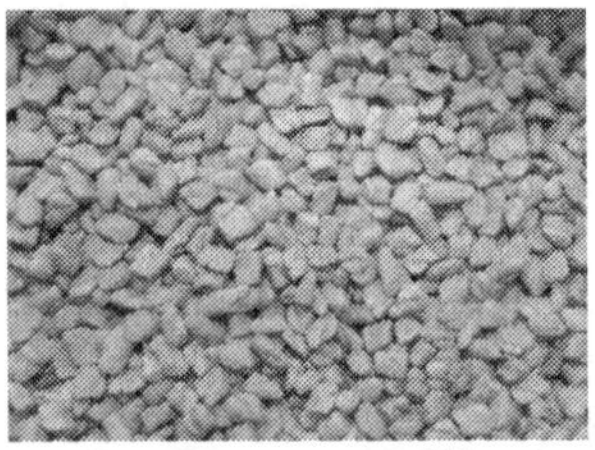

Fenugreek has been recognized as a medicinal plant for centuries. The Egyptians, Greeks and Romans used the aromatic seeds extensively. It was a stable included in the diet of Harem woman to increase the size and roundness of their breasts. Modern herbalists use fenugreek for nursing mothers to improve milk supply. Powdered seeds mixed with water or oil make a soothing paste that can be used as a skin emollient. Taken internally, fenugreek tea, capsules or tincture helps to stabilize blood sugar, and is considered an aphrodisiac. The rich combination of nutrients in Fenugreek include choline and trimethylamine (a sex hormone in frogs), Vitamins A, B 2, B 6, B 12, D, and essential oils. The aromatic compounds in the fenugreek seeds have a maple-syrup like odor, which freshens the breath.

Dosage: Tea- 1 tsp seed in 1 cup hot water, steep five minutes, 1-3 cups/day

Tincture/Extract- 10 drops 2X/day

Capsules- 500mg 2X/day

Poultice- soak ground seeds in enough hot water to make a paste, mix with Oil. Apply to skin

Caution: No adverse effects are known. However, if too much is used during nursing, the urine of mother and child may start to have a maple syrup odor, and could potentially lead to a misdiagnosis of 'maple syrup urine disease.'

Ginseng (*Panax Ginseng)*

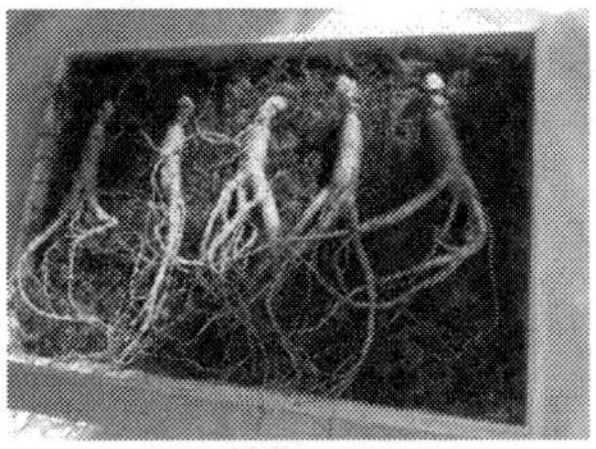

The name 'ginseng' is used to refer to several plant species. The three most common are *Panax Ginseng*- called Chinese or Korean Ginseng, *Panax quinqufolia*- American Ginseng and *Eleuthrococcus senticosis*- Siberian Ginseng. Ginseng confers a youthful vigor to men and women alike, for overall vitality and virility. The human-shaped root has been called 'man with thighs spread apart' by Native Americans. The Greek root word 'panacea' is reflected in the name 'panax' because of the wide rage of healings effects attributed to this root. Current studies conclude "Mean International Index of Erectile Function scores were significantly higher in patients treated with Korean red ginseng than in those who received placebo." (Hong B, Ji YH, Hong JH, Nam KY, Ahn TY, A double-blind crossover study evaluating the efficacy of korean red ginseng in patients with erectile dysfunction: a preliminary report., Journal of Urology, 2002, hNov;168(5):2027-3)

Dosage: 500-600 mg per day

Cautions: Ginseng Over Use Syndrome may produce symptoms of insomnia, irritability, anxiety, and heart palpitations, probably due to heightened testosterone levels. These effects are rare, and most often seen in young men using too much ginseng- probably because they already have enough testosterone!

Horny Goat Weed *(Epimedium grandiflorum)*

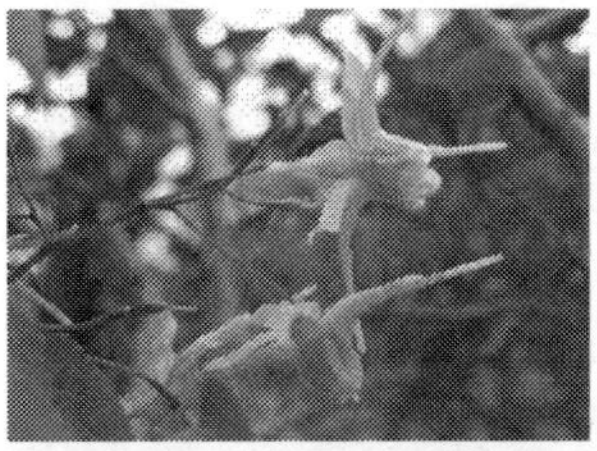

According to legend, a goat herder noticed that whenever his goats ate this herb, it revved up their sexual activity tremendously! The Chinese name for Epimedium, *Yin Yang Hua*, reflects the effect it has on both women (yin energy) and men (yang energy). Research suggests that this herb can

increase sperm count and semen density in men, and supports adrenal hormone production in both sexes. (Xiao Yong Xin. "A Pharmacological Study of Wu Zi Zhuang Yang Tang," Part 1, *Journal of Pharmacology and Clinical Practice of Traditional Chinese Medicine*, 1989, 5 (2):21. Also Part 11, 5 (5): 34. How *Yin Yang Huo* acts as a sexual hormonal stimulant.) It also improves circulation and has anti-fatigue properties. It is widely used as an aphrodisiac to increase sexual desire and activity.

Dosage: 500mg –1000mg/ day

Cautions: No known adverse affects.

(Ho/He) Shou Wu *(Polygonum multiflorum)*

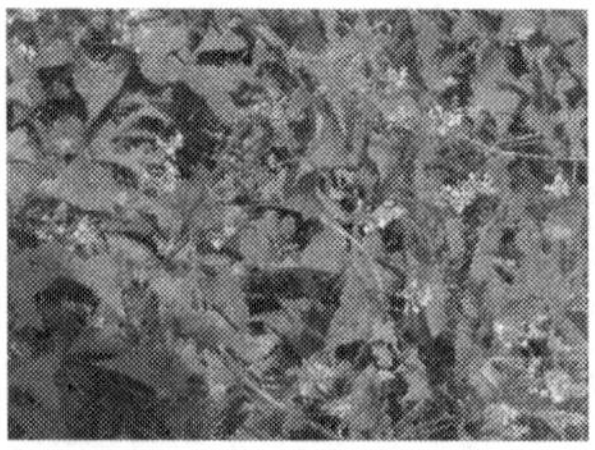

Ho Shou Wu is usually called **Fo-Ti** in the US. In China, it is revered for its mysterious properties of rejuvenation and anti-aging, and has been used for over 1000 years as a 'royal tonic' that nourishes the blood, cleanses the liver and kidneys, supports the joints, ligaments, tendons, muscles and sinews, increases the Chi energy of the liver and kidneys, enhances sexuality and fertility in both women and men. According to legend, it has the unique ability to return grey hair to its natural color. The name He Shou Wu translates to 'Mr. He's Black Hair tonic', or 'King He's White Hair Turned Black'. Chinese Legends describe a sickly, middle aged, infertile man named He, who discovered this herb and reversed the aging process. He fathered many children into old age, and turned his gray hair back to jet black!

Dosage : 5-10 pills, 3 X/ day

Cautions: May have a slight laxative effect. One case of liver toxicity has been reported. (Park GJ, Mann SP, Ngu MC., Acute hepatitis induced by Shou-Wu-Pian, a herbal product derived from Polygonum multiflorum. J Gastroenterol Hepatol 2001 Jan;16(1):115-7)

Kava kava(*Piper methysticum)*

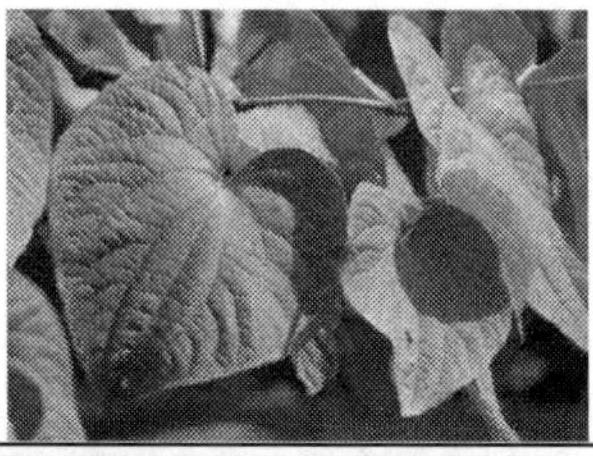

Kava kava grows in the South Pacific Islands and in the US in Hawaii. It is a wide-leafed vine, relative to the pepper plant. The part of the plant used to make the medicinal extract is the large root or rhizome. It has been used for thousands of years.

Captain Cook described its use in 1768 during one of his South Sea voyages. Kava is used to relax the body and mind, produce a tranquil state, enhance sociability and friendliness, and ease pain. It is touted as an aphrodisiac for women, although it may produce enough muscular relaxation to interfere with an erection in men. The most common use of Kava in western medicine is as an anti-anxiety agent. The active ingredients in Kava include kava lactones. Traditional use of Kava involves pounding the fresh root into a pulp, and then cooking it into a thick tea or soup. It is often served in a coconut shell. The Kava drink tastes bitter and causes a tingling sensation on the tongue and throat. It is available in the Health Food Store as a prepared Extract or Capsule, and may be standardized to contain 30-50% Kava lactones.

Dosage: Tea: 2-3 cups
Extract: 20 drops
Capsules: 100 mg

Cautions: High doses of Kava over extended periods of time can cause a rough skin condition called Kava dermatitis. It is reversible if Kava is discontinued. Kava can change the way you feel. When first using Kava do not drive or operate heavy machinery. Try it first in the evening, before a lovemaking session. There are a limited number of cases of liver toxicity that may be linked to kava use.

Lychii Fruit *(Lycium barbarum)*

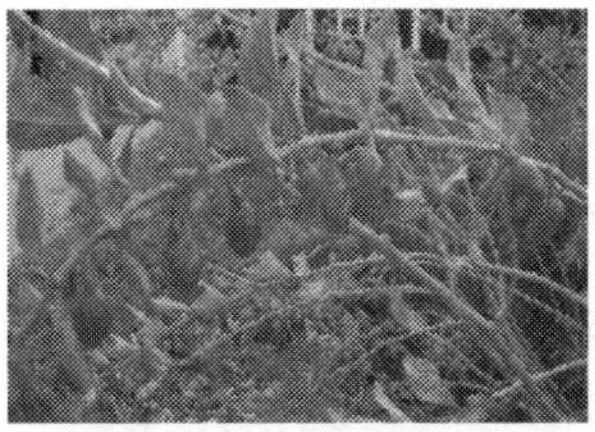

Lychii fruit, also called Wolfberry, and *Go-Qi-Zi,* has traditionally been used in China for thousands of years for its rejuvenating effects on sexuality and fertility. Lychii is a small red berry which is usually dried and prepared as a tea. Scientific studies have found that chemicals known as polysaccharides found in Lychii fruit protect both male and female sex organs from free radical damage. (Wang Y, Zhao H, Sheng X , et al., Protective effect of Fructus Lycii polysaccharides against time and hyperthermia-induced damage in cultured seminiferous epithelium., J Ethnopharmacol 2002 Oct;82(2-3):169-75) (Zhang B, Zhang X, Li W., The injury of Xenopus laevis oocytes membrane and its acetylcholine receptor by free radical and the protection of lycium barbarum polysaccharide, Zhongguo Ying Yong Sheng Li Xue Za Zhi 1997 Nov;13(4):322-5) Consuming lychii may increase testosterone levels which enhance libido and sexual function.

Dosage: ¼- ½ cup of Lychii berries soaked in one cup warm water/ day

Cautions: no adverse effects known

Maca (*Lepidium meyenii*)

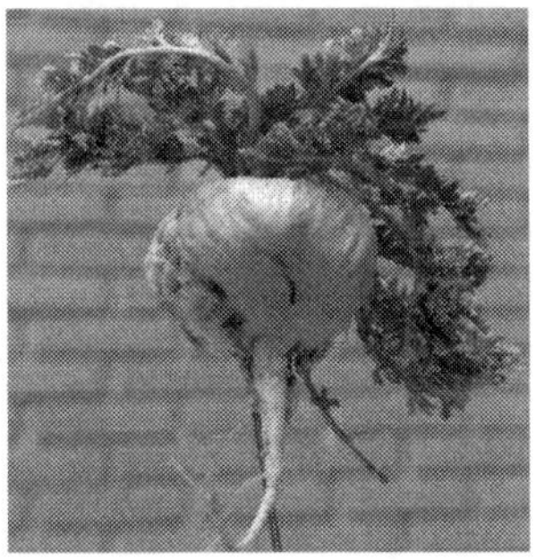

Maca is a cruciferous vegetable like Kale and Broccoli, that grows in the Andes Mountains in Peru. Native people dig up the root-like tuber and brew it into a strong drink. Both men and women partake of this brew shortly before going off in couples for connubial enjoyment. Incan warriors used maca before battle to increase strength and endurance. Science collaborates what these people have known for centuries, because showed a significant increase in sexual function in laboratory studies. (Bo Lin Zheng, Kan He, Calvin Hyungchan Kim, et al., **Effect of a lipidic extract from *Lepidium meyenii* on sexual behavior in mice and rats,** Urology, April 2000, Vol 55: 4,598-602) Maca is high in essential fatty acids, minerals such as phosphorus, calcium, magnesium and zinc, along with vitamins B, C and E, various phytosterols, and other nutritional factors known for their importance to sexual function.

Dosage: 300 mg

Cautions: no known adverse effects

Muira Puama *(Ptychopetalum olacoides)*

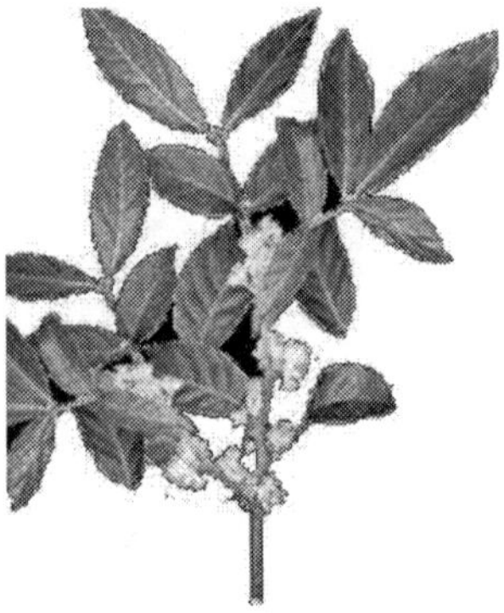

Muira puama is known as 'Warrior Wood" and " Potency Wood", and is used by the people of the northern Amazon area in Brazil for many health issues. It is considered a tonic for the neuromuscular system, (da Silva AL, Bardini S, Nunes DS, Elisabetsky E., Anxiogenic properties of Ptychopetalum olacoides Benth. (Marapuama), Phytother Res 2002 May;16(3):223-6} and helps with joint pains, menstrual cramps, PMS symptoms and mental disturbance. The entire plant is used in medicinal preparations, and contains sterols, including beta-sitosterol, which may account for its activity as a sexual stimulant. Muira Puama is listed in the British Herbal Pharmacopoeia for the treatment of impotence. In Brazil , it is used by both men and women to increase virility and vitality. Studies in France have verified its usefulness for men for both increased libido and impotence.

Dosage: 500 mg

Cautions: no known adverse effects

Oats *(Avena sativa)*

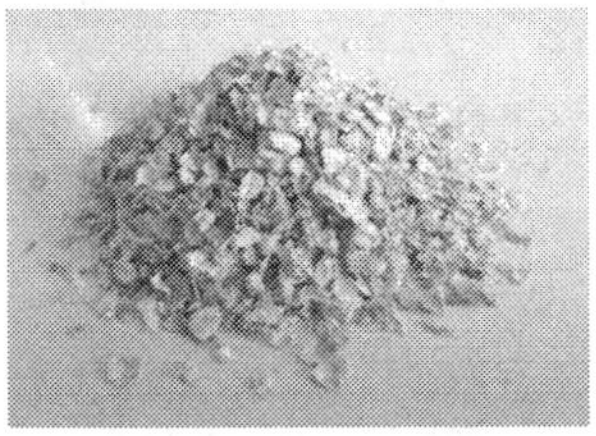

Oats are extremely high in nutrition, and can be added to the diet regularly, or used as an herbal supplement. Oats contain proteins, minerals, sterols including beta-sitosterol and beta-glucans, which enhance immune function, Vit B-complex and Vit E . The high fiber content has been touted by conventional medicine and Madison Ave alike to be cancer-protective. Oats provide 'nerve food' which offsets the effects of stress. It is helpful for depression, anxiety, reduced sex drive, fatigue and convalescing from illness or childbirth. Oats are also part of a heart healthy program when reduction of blood cholesterol is desired. Their high nutrient content helps the body form hormones efficiently, by supporting the glands, including the thyroid, adrenal, uterus, ovaries and testicles. The saying 'Sowing your wild oats' refers to the use of oats to increase vitality. When oats are soaked, they release a white-milky fluid which mirrors the appearance of sexual fluids. Oats are also useful externally on the skin for itching, rashes, and improvement of the complexion.

Dosage: a bowl of oatmeal a day (Choose organic oats if possible)
Tincture/Extract- 10-20 ml 2X/day
Capsules 500-1000 mg 2X/day
Bath – heat 1 qt of water with one cup of oats or a handful of oatstraw.

Cautions: People with gluten sensitivities may cross-react to oats

Quebracho *(Aspidosperma quebracho-blanco)*

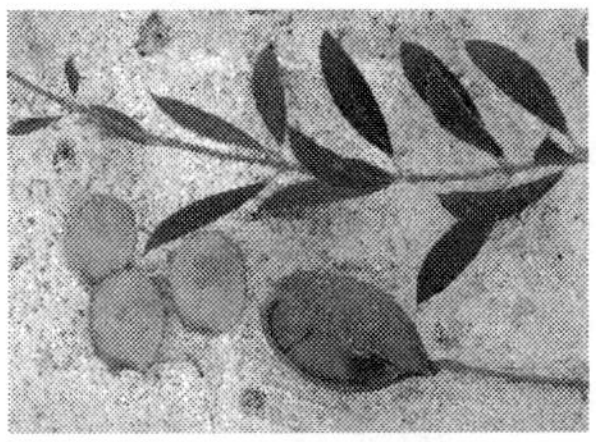

Quebracho is an evergreen tree which grows in South America, where is has been used traditionally by native people. It was introduced into Europe as a medicine in 1878. Quebracho has been used for fevers, blocked circulation and respiratory problems such as asthma. The bark of the tree is

the part used as medicine. Quebracho's influence on improving circulation may be the action that has aphrodisiac properties, by allowing blood to freely flow to the sex organs. The tea has a very bitter taste, so it may be easier to use quebracho in capsule form.

Dosage: 1-2ml of fluid extract 2 X per day
250mg capsules 2X per day

Cautions: No adverse effects known. Quebracho is generally recognized as safe by the FDA. May be contraindicated for High Blood Pressure.

Sarsaparilla (*Smilax officinalis, spec.)*

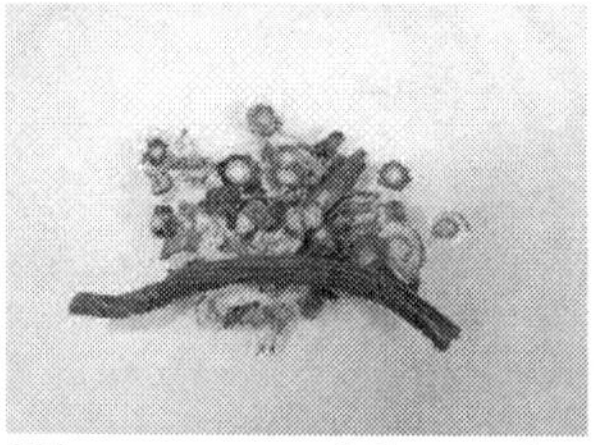

The name "Sarsaparilla" is derived from the Spanish word, *Sarza* for bramble, and *parilla* for vine. During the 1500's, Sarsaparilla was used extensively to treat syphilis, and other STD's (sexually transmitted diseases). It was used by men who frequented brothels to try to avoid catching these illnesses, although the effectiveness for this use is questionable. Sarsaparilla is best known in the US as the flavoring agent in root beer, although its medicinal use touted overall tonic properties for a wide variety of ailments. Sarsaparilla is rich in nutrients including calcium, iron, iodine, manganese, potassium, sulfur, Vitamins B, A , C and D, and contains active constituents that may help to increase hormones including testosterone and progesterone, and has been attributed with increased virility in men and desire in women.

Dosage: Brewed as a tea- 1-2 cups per day
500mg/ 2 times per day

Cautions: The German Commission E monograph warns that excessive use of Sarsaparilla (*many times the recommended dosage*) may cause stomach and kidney irritation

Saw Palmetto *(Serenoa repens)*

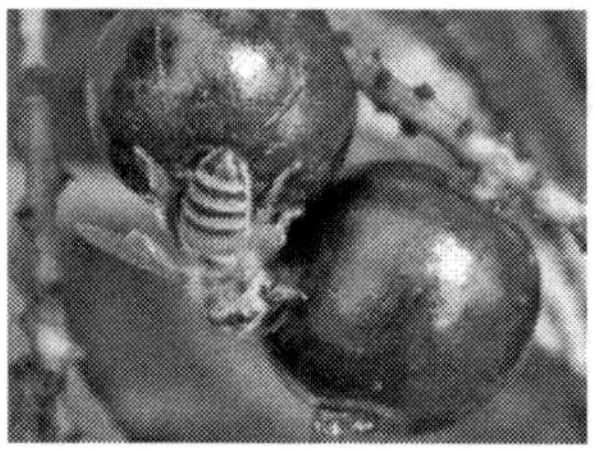

Saw Palmetto has been used as a medicinal plant for centuries by the Seminole Indians in Florida, and can also be traced back to the Mayan Civilization. Native People knew that the saw palmetto berries were ripe and ready, when they noticed that the local deer and other animals were looking sleek and sassy. The berries of this dwarf palm tree are high in fatty acid sterols which have been scientifically studied for their positive effect on reducing BPH (benign prostatic hypertrophy) in men, and have also been used to enhance breast size in women. Traditionally, saw palmetto is considered a sexual tonic for both men and women.

Dosage: ½ cup fresh or dried Saw Palmetto berries per day
80- 320 mg 2 times per day
160 mg , (standardized to 80-90% fatty acid sterols) 2 X per day- common dose

Cautions: No adverse effects have been reported. There is some concern that measuring PSA may be interfered with during Saw Palmetto use, but this is controversial.

Tribulus *(Tribulus terrestes)*

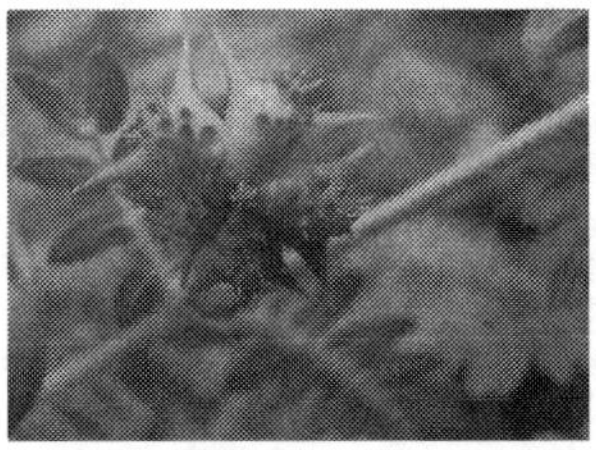

Tribulus is a brownish fruit has been used for thousands of years, in the Indian traditional healing system, called Ayurveda. It is effective for both men and women to help increase vitality. In men, it helps to reverse impotence and increase sperm count, while activating desire in both sexes, possibly by increasing testosterone levels.

Dosage: 500mg/ day

Cautions: none known

Yohimbe *(Pausinystalia yohimbe)*

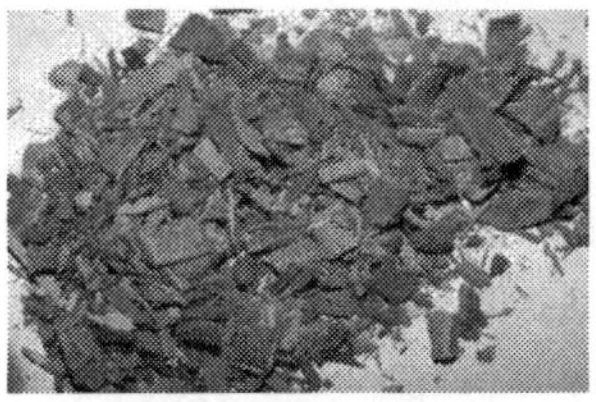

Yohimbe is derived from bark stripped from a tall evergreen West African tree. In its native land Yohimbe may be made into a tea, smoked, or processed into a powder and sniffed. In the western world, *yohimbine*, the primary active constituent of yohimbe, is also available as a prescription drug, *yohimbine hydrochloride*, used for erectile dysfunction. (Ernst E, Pittler MH. Yohimbine for erectile dysfunction: A systematic review and meta-analysis of randomized clinical trials. *J Urol* 1998;159:433–6) Yohimbe increases testosterone blood levels in both men and women, causing enhanced sex drive. It also stimulates circulation. This is especially helpful for men with decreased pelvic circulation, and may offset vaginal atrophy in women.

Dosage: Dosage is important with this herb. A safe amount is 15-30 mg/ day. Stick to the label directions on the product you are using.

Cautions: Do not use with kidney or liver disease, high blood pressure, or heart arrhythmias. Possible side effects include anxiety, increased blood pressure, and facial hair growth in women. These side effects are infrequent and reversible. It is interesting to note that some people who experience these effects with the herbal extract often have no problem taking the prescription drug! The active ingredients in yohimbine can block the action of the drug brimonidine.

Zallouh *(Ferulis harmonis)*

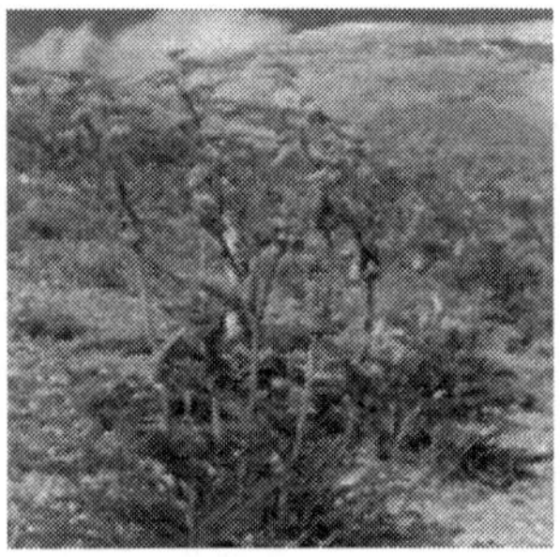

Zallouh grows in the Middle East, and is harvested and sold as a plant based aphrodisiac by the Syrian Army. The root of this plant has been used as an anti-aging vitality enhancer in traditional folk medicine for centuries. It not only aids those who are experiencing low libido, but has also been reported to increase lust in healthy men and women. Recent clinical trials validate the efficacy of Zallouh root as a treatment for erectile dysfunction. This herb contains ferulic acid and probably works by dilating blood vessels and stimulating circulation.

Dosage: 400mg- 800mg

Cautions: may increase blood pressure; causes flushing and headache in some users

<u>Herbal Vitality Aphrodisiac Recipe</u>

You can prepare a simple Vitality and Virility combination by using the herbs listed below. Purchase liquid extracts, available in most health food stores.

Ginseng Extract
Ginger Extract
Oat Extract
Damiana Extract

Muira Puama Extract
Passionflower Extract

Combine 20 drops of each herb in ¼ cup of warm water; add ½ ounce of Amaretto or some other flavored liquor. Relax and enjoy!

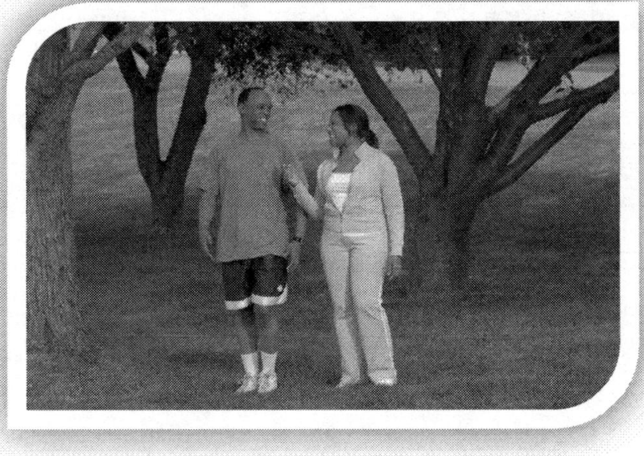

Image credits:

Elderly couple dancing – By maveric2003
http://www.everystockphoto.com/photographer.php?photographer_id=468

Damiana - By Nordschitz (Own work) [CC BY-SA 4.0 (http://creativecommons.org/licenses/by-sa/4.0)], via Wikimedia Commons

Licorice root - By KoS (Own work) [Public domain], via Wikimedia Commons

Deer Antlers - By Red_deer_stag.jpg: Mehmet Karatay derivative work: Mehmet Karatay (Red_deer_stag.jpg) [CC BY-SA 3.0 (http://creativecommons.org/licenses/by-sa/3.0) or GFDL (http://www.gnu.org/copyleft/fdl.html)], via Wikimedia Commons

Horny Goat Weed - By Sphl (Photo taken by Sphl.) [GFDL (http://www.gnu.org/copyleft/fdl.html), CC-BY-SA-3.0 (http://creativecommons.org/licenses/by-sa/3.0/), CC BY-SA 2.5 (http://creativecommons.org/licenses/by-sa/2.5) or CC BY-SA 2.1 jp (http://creativecommons.org/licenses/by-sa/2.1/jp/deed.en)], via Wikimedia Commons

Ho/He Shou Wu/ Polygonum Multiflorum - "Fallopia multiflora leaf" by I, Doronenko. Licensed under CC BY 2.5 via Commons - https://commons.wikimedia.org/wiki/File:Fallopia_multiflora_leaf.jpg#/media/File:Fallopia_multiflora_leaf.jpg

Kava kava(Piper methysticum) - "Starr 070515-7054 Piper methysticum" by Forest & Kim Starr. Licensed under CC BY 3.0 via Commons -

https://commons.wikimedia.org/wiki/File:Starr_070515-7054_Piper_methysticum.jpg#/media/File:Starr_070515-7054_Piper_methysticum.jpg

Lychii fruit/Wolfberries - "Lycium-barbarum-fruits" by Sten Porse - Self-published work by Sten Porse. Licensed under CC BY-SA 3.0 via Commons - https://commons.wikimedia.org/wiki/File:Lycium-barbarum-fruits.JPG#/media/File:Lycium-barbarum-fruits.JPG

Maca – By http://focoemvidasaudavel.blogspot.com/2013/11/maca-dos-andes-aumenta-libido-melhora.html

Polygonum Multiflorum by Fanghong (Own work) [GFDL (http://www.gnu.org/copyleft/fdl.html), CC-BY-SA-3.0 (http://creativecommons.org/licenses/by-sa/3.0/) or CC BY-SA 1.0 (http://creativecommons.org/licenses/by-sa/1.0)], via Wikimedia Commons

Quebracho - By Dick Culbert from Gibsons, B.C., Canada (Aspidosperma quebracho-blanco) [CC BY 2.0 (http://creativecommons.org/licenses/by/2.0)], via Wikimedia Commons

Sarsaparilla - By Maša Sinreih in Valentina Vivod (Own work) [CC BY-SA 3.0 (http://creativecommons.org/licenses/by-sa/3.0) or GFDL (http://www.gnu.org/copyleft/fdl.html)], via Wikimedia Commons

Saw Palmetto Berries - By Bob Peterson from North Palm Beach, Florida, Planet Earth! [CC BY-SA 2.0 (http://creativecommons.org/licenses/by-sa/2.0)], via Wikimedia Commons

Tribulus - Forest & Kim Starr [CC BY 3.0 (http://creativecommons.org/licenses/by/3.0)], via Wikimedia Commons

Yohimbe Bark - http://yohimbebark.wikispaces.com/Yohimbe+Bark

"Salt lassi" by Raksanand - Own work. Licensed under CC BY-SA 4.0 via Commons - https://commons.wikimedia.org/wiki/File:Salt_lassi.jpg#/media/File:Salt_lassi.jpg

Zallouh plants - http://www.medicinehunter.com/zallouh

DISCLAIMER: THIS Ebook DOES NOT PROVIDE MEDICAL ADVICE

The information, including but not limited to, text, graphics, images and other material contained in this Ebook are for informational purposes only. The purpose of this Ebook is to promote broad consumer understanding and knowledge of various health topics. It is not intended to be a substitute for professional medical advice, diagnosis or treatment. Always seek the advice of your physician or other qualified health care provider with any questions you may have regarding a medical condition or treatment and before undertaking a new health care regimen, and never disregard professional medical advice or delay in seeking it because of something you have read on in this Ebook. The author takes no responsibility and shall not be held liable for any effects or adverse effects that may occur due to the use of any information that the reader chooses to use from this publication.

Made in the USA
Monee, IL
08 November 2026

67378651R00015